LOW FIBER DIET COOKBOOK

FOR DIVERTICULITIS

Delicious Recipes for Managing Diverticulitis

T. John

COPYRIGHT PAGE

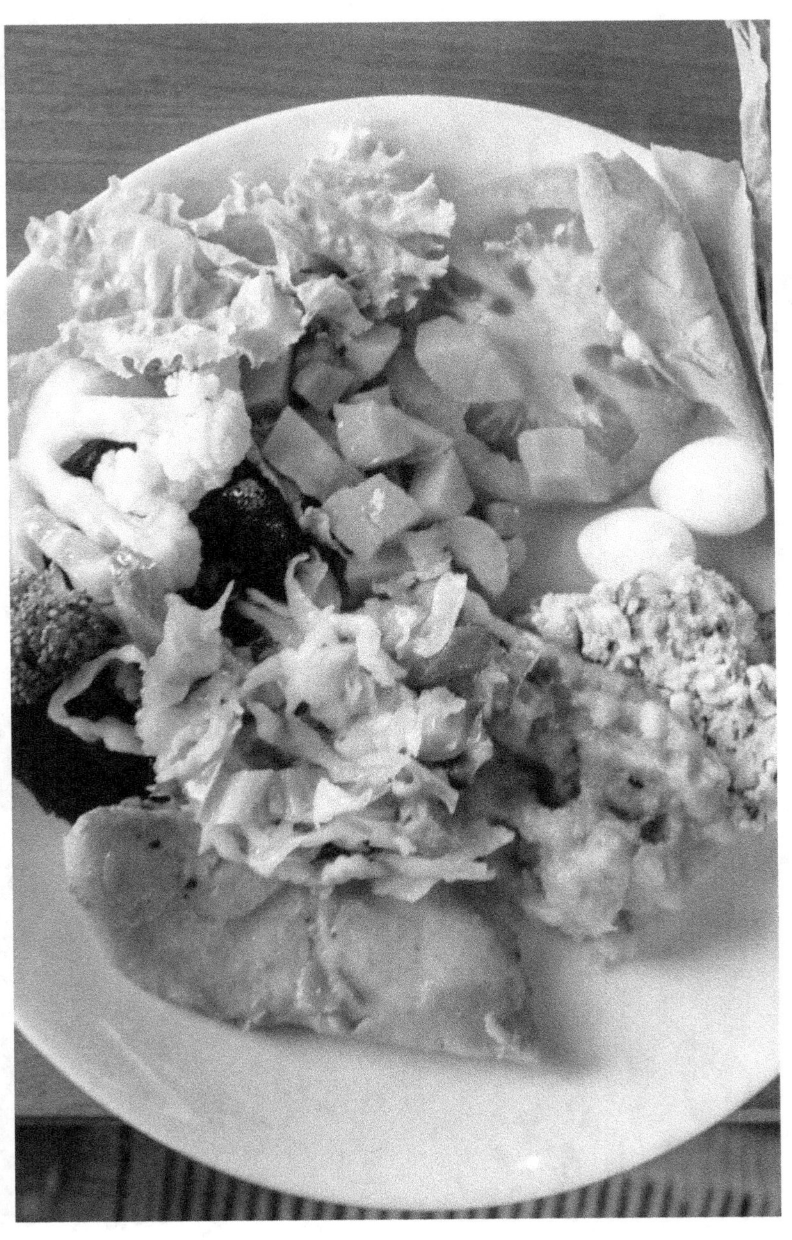

TABLE OF CONTENTS

Chapter 3: Lunch Recipes 40

Chapter 4: Dinner Recipes 55

Chapter 5: Snacks and Appetizers 71

CONCLUSION 109

INTRODUCTION

Diverticulitis is a medical condition characterized by the inflammation or infection of small pouches called diverticula that develop in the lining of the digestive tract, particularly in the colon. These diverticula are formed when weak spots in the colon's muscular walls allow the inner lining to protrude through. While diverticula themselves do not cause symptoms, complications can arise if they become inflamed or infected, leading to diverticulitis.

Understanding a Low Fiber Diet

A low fiber diet, also known as a low-residue diet, is commonly recommended for individuals with diverticulitis. The primary goal of this dietary approach is to minimize the strain on the digestive system and provide relief from symptoms by reducing the volume and bulk of stool. A low fiber diet limits the intake of foods that are high in fiber, such as whole grains, fruits, vegetables, and legumes, as these can be difficult to digest and may aggravate the inflamed diverticula.

Benefits of a Low Fiber Diet for Diverticulitis

Adhering to a low fiber diet can offer several benefits for individuals with diverticulitis. Firstly, it helps to alleviate the symptoms associated with the condition, including abdominal pain, cramping, bloating, and changes in bowel movements. By reducing the amount of fiber passing through the intestines, the workload on the digestive system is decreased, allowing the inflamed diverticula to heal and preventing further irritation.

Secondly, a low fiber diet promotes the rest and recovery of the digestive system. The reduced intake of high-fiber foods gives the digestive organs a break and allows them to heal. This can be particularly beneficial during acute flare-ups of diverticulitis when the colon needs time to recuperate.

Additionally, a low fiber diet may help prevent complications, such as diverticular bleeding or perforation. By minimizing the strain on the diverticula, the risk of these complications can be reduced. However, it is important to note that a low fiber diet is typically recommended for short-term use during acute episodes of diverticulitis and should not be followed long-term without medical supervision.

Tips for Following a Low Fiber Diet

Successfully adhering to a low fiber diet requires careful planning and consideration of food choices. Here are some tips to help you navigate this dietary approach:

1. Limit high-fiber foods: Avoid or minimize the consumption of foods that are high in fiber, such as whole grains, fruits, vegetables, nuts, and seeds. Instead, focus on low-fiber alternatives.

2. Choose refined grains: Opt for refined grains like white bread, white rice, and refined pasta, which have had the fiber-rich bran and germ removed.

3. Include low-fiber fruits and vegetables: While most fruits and vegetables are restricted on a low fiber diet, certain low-fiber options can still be enjoyed, such as peeled and cooked fruits, canned fruits in juice, and well-cooked or canned vegetables.

4. Consume lean protein: Incorporate lean protein sources into your meals, such as skinless poultry, fish, eggs, and tofu. These provide essential nutrients without adding excessive fiber.

5. Cook foods thoroughly: Ensure that foods are cooked until they are soft and tender, as this aids in digestion and reduces the strain on the digestive system.

6. Stay hydrated: Drink an adequate amount of fluids throughout the day to prevent dehydration and aid in digestion. Aim for at least eight glasses of water daily unless advised otherwise by your healthcare provider.

7. Keep a food diary: Keeping a record of your meals and symptoms can help identify trigger foods or patterns that may worsen your symptoms. This can assist in fine-tuning your diet and making necessary adjustments.

8. Consult a healthcare professional: It is essential to consult with a healthcare professional, such as a registered dietitian or gastroenterologist, before starting a low fiber diet. They can provide

personalized guidance based on your specific needs and medical history.

How to Use This Cookbook

This cookbook has been carefully crafted to provide you with a wide range of delicious and satisfying recipes that comply with a low fiber diet. The chapters are organized in a logical and practical manner to assist you in planning and preparing meals that are both nourishing and gentle on your digestive system.

Before diving into the recipes, take the time to read through the entire cookbook to familiarize yourself with the chapters and the meal plan provided. The 30-day meal plan in Chapter 2 offers a comprehensive guide for your dietary journey, ensuring that you have a balanced and varied selection of meals throughout the month.

Chapters 2 to 7 contain a diverse collection of recipes, each carefully developed to be flavorful, easy to digest, and suitable for a low fiber diet. Whether you're looking for breakfast ideas, lunch and dinner options, snacks and appetizers, desserts, or refreshing smoothies, you will find a plethora of choices to satisfy your taste buds while adhering to the dietary guidelines.

Chapter 1: 30 Day Meal Plan

This 30-day meal plan provides a variety of options for breakfast, lunch, dinner, snacks, desserts, and smoothies. Feel free to repeat the plan or mix and match the recipes based on your preferences and dietary needs.

Week 1: Meal Plan and Recipes

Day 1:

Breakfast: Scrambled Eggs with Spinach and Tomatoes

Lunch: Chicken and Vegetable Stir-Fry

Dinner: Grilled Chicken Breast with Steamed Vegetables

Snack: Greek Yogurt Dip with Fresh Veggies

Dessert: Banana "Ice Cream" with Almonds

Smoothie: Berry Blast Smoothie

Day 2:

Breakfast: Oatmeal with Apples and Cinnamon

Lunch: Turkey and Avocado Wrap

Dinner: Baked Cod with Herbed Quinoa

Snack: Avocado Hummus with Rice Crackers

Dessert: Baked Apples with Cinnamon and Yogurt

Smoothie: Tropical Green Smoothie

Day 3:

Breakfast: Yogurt Parfait with Berries and Nuts

Lunch: Tuna Salad Lettuce Wraps

Dinner: Beef and Broccoli Stir-Fry

Snack: Baked Sweet Potato Fries

Dessert: Chocolate Avocado Pudding

Smoothie: Banana and Peanut Butter Smoothie

Day 4:

Breakfast: Vegetable Frittata

Lunch: Shrimp and Quinoa Salad

Dinner: Turkey Meatballs with Marinara Sauce

Snack: Caprese Skewers with Balsamic Glaze

Dessert: Berry Parfait with Greek Yogurt

Smoothie: Spinach and Mango Smoothie

Day 5:

Breakfast: Banana Pancakes

Lunch: Baked Salmon with Lemon and Herbs

Dinner: Stuffed Bell Peppers with Ground Turkey

Snack: Deviled Eggs with Pickles

Dessert: Coconut Macaroons

Smoothie: Chocolate Banana Protein Smoothie

Day 6:

Breakfast: Smooth Peanut Butter Toast

Lunch: Egg Salad with Greek Yogurt

Dinner: Lemon Herb Roasted Chicken Thighs

Snack: Guacamole with Carrot Sticks

Dessert: Chia Seed Pudding with Mango

Smoothie: Blueberry and Almond Smoothie

Day 7:

Breakfast: Quinoa Breakfast Bowl

Lunch: Lentil Soup with Carrots and Celery

Dinner: Shrimp Scampi with Zucchini Noodles

Snack: Roasted Chickpeas with Herbs

Dessert: Poached Pears with Honey and Cinnamon

Smoothie: Avocado and Spinach Smoothie

Week 2: Meal Plan and Recipes

Day 8:

Breakfast: Egg and Vegetable Muffins

Lunch: Greek Salad with Grilled Chicken

Dinner: Vegetable Curry with Brown Rice

Snack: Spinach and Artichoke Dip

Dessert: Lemon Bars with Almond Flour Crust

Smoothie: Pineapple and Coconut Smoothie

Day 9:

Breakfast: Blueberry Chia Pudding

Lunch: Zucchini Noodles with Tomato Sauce

Dinner: Pork Tenderloin with Roasted Vegetables

Snack: Cucumber and Cream Cheese Roll-Ups

Dessert: Pumpkin Muffins with Walnuts

Smoothie: Strawberry and Oat Smoothie

Day 10:

Breakfast: Rice Porridge with Raisins

Lunch: Roasted Vegetable and Quinoa Salad

Dinner: Teriyaki Tofu Stir-Fry

Snack: Sliced Apple with Almond Butter

Dessert: Grilled Pineapple with Coconut Whipped Cream

Smoothie: Peach and Greek Yogurt Smoothie

Day 11:

Breakfast: Scrambled Eggs with Spinach and Tomatoes

Lunch: Chicken and Vegetable Stir-Fry

Dinner: Grilled Chicken Breast with Steamed Vegetables

Snack: Greek Yogurt Dip with Fresh Veggies

Dessert: Banana "Ice Cream" with Almonds

Smoothie: Berry Blast Smoothie

Day 12:

Breakfast: Oatmeal with Apples and Cinnamon

Lunch: Turkey and Avocado Wrap

Dinner: Baked Cod with Herbed Quinoa

Snack: Avocado Hummus with Rice Crackers

Dessert: Baked Apples with Cinnamon and Yogurt

Smoothie: Tropical Green Smoothie

Day 13:

Breakfast: Yogurt Parfait with Berries and Nuts

Lunch: Tuna Salad Lettuce Wraps

Dinner: Beef and Broccoli Stir-Fry

Snack: Baked Sweet Potato Fries

Dessert: Chocolate Avocado Pudding

Smoothie: Banana and Peanut Butter Smoothie

Day 14:

Breakfast: Vegetable Frittata

Lunch: Shrimp and Quinoa Salad

Dinner: Turkey Meatballs with Marinara Sauce

Snack: Caprese Skewers with Balsamic Glaze

Dessert: Berry Parfait with Greek Yogurt

Smoothie: Spinach and Mango Smoothie

Week 3: Meal Plan and Recipes

Day 15:

Breakfast: Banana Pancakes

Lunch: Baked Salmon with Lemon and Herbs

Dinner: Stuffed Bell Peppers with Ground Turkey

Snack: Deviled Eggs with Pickles

Dessert: Coconut Macaroons

Smoothie: Chocolate Banana Protein Smoothie

Day 16:

Breakfast: Smooth Peanut Butter Toast

Lunch: Egg Salad with Greek Yogurt

Dinner: Lemon Herb Roasted Chicken Thighs

Snack: Guacamole with Carrot Sticks

Dessert: Chia Seed Pudding with Mango

Smoothie: Blueberry and Almond Smoothie

Day 17:

Breakfast: Quinoa Breakfast Bowl

Lunch: Lentil Soup with Carrots and Celery

Dinner: Shrimp Scampi with Zucchini Noodles

Snack: Roasted Chickpeas with Herbs

Dessert: Poached Pears with Honey and Cinnamon

Smoothie: Avocado and Spinach Smoothie

Day 18:

Breakfast: Egg and Vegetable Muffins

Lunch: Greek Salad with Grilled Chicken

Dinner: Vegetable Curry with Brown Rice

Snack: Spinach and Artichoke Dip

Dessert: Lemon Bars with Almond Flour Crust

Smoothie: Pineapple and Coconut Smoothie

Day 19:

Breakfast: Blueberry Chia Pudding

Lunch: Zucchini Noodles with Tomato Sauce

Dinner: Pork Tenderloin with Roasted Vegetables

Snack: Cucumber and Cream Cheese Roll-Ups

Dessert: Pumpkin Muffins with Walnuts

Smoothie: Strawberry and Oat Smoothie

Day 20:

Breakfast: Rice Porridge with Raisins

Lunch: Roasted Vegetable and Quinoa Salad

Dinner: Teriyaki Tofu Stir-Fry

Snack: Sliced Apple with Almond Butter

Dessert: Grilled Pineapple with Coconut Whipped Cream

Smoothie: Peach and Greek Yogurt Smoothie

Day 21:

Breakfast: Scrambled Eggs with Spinach and Tomatoes

Lunch: Chicken and Vegetable Stir-Fry

Dinner: Grilled Chicken Breast with Steamed Vegetables

Snack: Greek Yogurt Dip with Fresh Veggies

Dessert: Banana "Ice Cream" with Almonds

Smoothie: Berry Blast Smoothie

Week 4: Meal Plan and Recipes

Day 22:

Breakfast: Oatmeal with Apples and Cinnamon

Lunch: Turkey and Avocado Wrap

Dinner: Baked Cod with Herbed Quinoa

Snack: Avocado Hummus with Rice Crackers

Dessert: Baked Apples with Cinnamon and Yogurt

Smoothie: Tropical Green Smoothie

Day 23:

Breakfast: Yogurt Parfait with Berries and Nuts

Lunch: Tuna Salad Lettuce Wraps

Dinner: Beef and Broccoli Stir-Fry

Snack: Baked Sweet Potato Fries

Dessert: Chocolate Avocado Pudding

Smoothie: Banana and Peanut Butter Smoothie

Day 24:

Breakfast: Vegetable Frittata

Lunch: Shrimp and Quinoa Salad

Dinner: Turkey Meatballs with Marinara Sauce

Snack: Caprese Skewers with Balsamic Glaze

Dessert: Berry Parfait with Greek Yogurt

Smoothie: Spinach and Mango Smoothie

Day 25:

Breakfast: Banana Pancakes

Lunch: Baked Salmon with Lemon and Herbs

Dinner: Stuffed Bell Peppers with Ground Turkey

Snack: Deviled Eggs with Pickles

Dessert: Coconut Macaroons

Smoothie: Chocolate Banana Protein Smoothie

Day 26:

Breakfast: Smooth Peanut Butter Toast

Lunch: Egg Salad with Greek Yogurt

Dinner: Lemon Herb Roasted Chicken Thighs

Snack: Guacamole with Carrot Sticks

Dessert: Chia Seed Pudding with Mango

Smoothie: Blueberry and Almond Smoothie

Day 27:

Breakfast: Quinoa Breakfast Bowl

Lunch: Lentil Soup with Carrots and Celery

Dinner: Shrimp Scampi with Zucchini Noodles

Snack: Roasted Chickpeas with Herbs

Dessert: Poached Pears with Honey and Cinnamon

Smoothie: Avocado and Spinach Smoothie

Day 28:

Breakfast: Egg and Vegetable Muffins

Lunch: Greek Salad with Grilled Chicken

Dinner: Vegetable Curry with Brown Rice

Snack: Spinach and Artichoke Dip

Dessert: Lemon Bars with Almond Flour Crust

Smoothie: Pineapple and Coconut Smoothie

Day 29:

Breakfast: Blueberry Chia Pudding

Lunch: Zucchini Noodles with Tomato Sauce

Dinner: Pork Tenderloin with Roasted Vegetables

Snack: Cucumber and Cream Cheese Roll-Ups

Dessert: Pumpkin Muffins with Walnuts

Smoothie: Strawberry and Oat Smoothie

Day 30:

Breakfast: Rice Porridge with Raisins

Lunch: Roasted Vegetable and Quinoa Salad

Dinner: Teriyaki Tofu Stir-Fry

Snack: Sliced Apple with Almond Butter

Dessert: Grilled Pineapple with Coconut Whipped Cream

Smoothie: Peach and Greek Yogurt Smoothie

Chapter 2: Breakfast Recipes

In this chapter, we will explore ten delicious and nutritious breakfast recipes that are suitable for a low fiber diet. These recipes are designed to provide you with a satisfying and wholesome start to your day while being gentle on your digestive system. Let's dive in and discover the flavors and textures that await you.

Scrambled Eggs with Spinach and Tomatoes

Ingredients:

- 2 eggs
- 1 cup fresh spinach leaves
- 1/2 cup cherry tomatoes, halved
- Salt and pepper to taste
- Cooking oil or butter for the pan

Instructions:

1. Heat a non-stick skillet over medium heat and add a small amount of cooking oil or butter.

2. In a bowl, whisk the eggs and season with salt and pepper.

3. Pour the beaten eggs into the skillet and gently scramble them with a spatula until they are almost cooked through.

4. Add the spinach leaves and cherry tomatoes to the skillet and continue cooking for another minute or until the spinach wilts and the tomatoes soften.

5. Remove from heat and transfer the scrambled eggs with spinach and tomatoes to a plate.

6. Serve hot and enjoy a nutrient-packed breakfast!

Oatmeal with Apples and Cinnamon

Ingredients:

- 1/2 cup rolled oats
- 1 cup water or milk (dairy or non-dairy)
- 1 small apple, peeled, cored, and diced
- 1/2 teaspoon cinnamon
- 1 tablespoon honey or maple syrup (optional)
- Nuts or seeds for topping (optional)

Instructions:

1. In a small saucepan, bring the water or milk to a
    boil.

2. Stir in the rolled oats and reduce the heat to low.

3. Cook the oats according to the package instructions,
    usually for about 5 minutes, stirring occasionally.

4. Once the oats have absorbed most of the liquid and
    reached your desired consistency, remove the
    saucepan from heat.

5. Add the diced apple, cinnamon, and honey or maple
    syrup if desired. Stir well to combine.

6. Transfer the oatmeal to a bowl and sprinkle with
    nuts or seeds for extra crunch and nutrition.

7. Let it cool for a minute or two before savoring the
    delightful flavors of this comforting breakfast.

Yogurt Parfait with Berries and Nuts

Ingredients:

- 1 cup low-fat yogurt (plain or flavored)
- 1/4 cup granola
- 1/4 cup mixed berries (such as strawberries,
  blueberries, and raspberries)

- 2 tablespoons chopped nuts (such as almonds, walnuts, or pecans)
- 1 tablespoon honey (optional)

Instructions:

1. Choose a glass or a bowl for layering your parfait.
2. Start by adding a spoonful of yogurt to the bottom of the glass.
3. Top the yogurt with a layer of granola, followed by a layer of mixed berries.
4. Repeat the layers until you reach the top of the glass, finishing with a dollop of yogurt.
5. Sprinkle the chopped nuts on top for added crunch and drizzle with honey if desired.
6. Serve immediately and relish the creamy texture, fruity sweetness, and nutty goodness of this delightful yogurt parfait.

Vegetable Frittata

Ingredients:

- 4 large eggs
- 1/4 cup milk (dairy or non-dairy)

- 1/2 cup chopped mixed vegetables (such as bell peppers, zucchini, and mushrooms)
- 1/4 cup shredded cheese (such as cheddar or mozzarella)
- Salt and pepper to taste
- Cooking oil or butter for the pan

Instructions:

1. Preheat your oven to 375°F (190°C).
2. In a bowl, whisk together the eggs, milk, salt, and pepper.
3. Heat an oven-safe skillet over medium heat and add a small amount of cooking oil or butter.
4. Sauté the mixed vegetables in the skillet until they are tender.
5. Pour the egg mixture over the sautéed vegetables and sprinkle the shredded cheese on top.
6. Transfer the skillet to the preheated oven and bake for approximately 15 minutes or until the frittata is set and slightly golden on top.

7. Remove from the oven and let it cool for a few minutes before slicing and serving this savory vegetable frittata.

Banana Pancakes

Ingredients:

- 1 ripe banana, mashed
- 2 eggs
- 1/4 cup oat flour or all-purpose flour
- 1/2 teaspoon baking powder
- 1/2 teaspoon vanilla extract
- Cooking oil or butter for the pan

Instructions:

1. In a bowl, combine the mashed banana, eggs, oat flour or all-purpose flour, baking powder, and vanilla extract. Mix until well combined.
2. Heat a non-stick skillet or griddle over medium heat and lightly grease it with cooking oil or butter.
3. Pour approximately 1/4 cup of the pancake batter onto the skillet for each pancake.

4. Cook until bubbles form on the surface of the pancake, then flip it and cook the other side until golden brown.

5. Repeat the process with the remaining batter, adding more oil or butter to the skillet as needed.

6. Serve the banana pancakes warm, and if desired, top them with sliced bananas, a drizzle of honey, or a sprinkle of cinnamon.

Smooth Peanut Butter Toast

Ingredients:

- 2 slices of bread (whole grain or white)
- 2 tablespoons smooth peanut butter
- Sliced banana (optional)
- Honey or maple syrup (optional)

Instructions:

1. Toast the bread slices until they are golden brown and crispy.

2. Spread the smooth peanut butter evenly on each slice of toast.

3. If desired, add a layer of sliced banana on top of the peanut butter.

4. For a touch of sweetness, drizzle honey or maple syrup over the toast.

5. Serve immediately and enjoy the delightful combination of nutty peanut butter, soft bread, and optional fruity sweetness.

Quinoa Breakfast Bowl

Ingredients:

- 1/2 cup cooked quinoa
- 1/4 cup low-fat yogurt (plain or flavored)
- 1/4 cup mixed berries (such as blueberries, strawberries, and raspberries)
- 1 tablespoon honey or maple syrup
- 1 tablespoon chopped nuts or seeds (such as almonds, walnuts, or chia seeds)

Instructions:

1. In a bowl, combine the cooked quinoa and low-fat yogurt. Mix well.

2. Top the quinoa and yogurt mixture with mixed berries.

3. Drizzle honey or maple syrup over the berries for natural sweetness.

4. Sprinkle the chopped nuts or seeds on top for added texture and nutrition.

5. Gently stir all the ingredients together and savor the delightful combination of flavors and textures in this wholesome quinoa breakfast bowl.

Egg and Vegetable Muffins

Ingredients:

- 4 eggs
- 1/4 cup milk (dairy or non-dairy)
- 1/2 cup chopped mixed vegetables (such as bell peppers, spinach, and onions)
- 1/4 cup shredded cheese (such as cheddar or feta)
- Salt and pepper to taste
- Cooking oil or butter for greasing the muffin tin

Instructions:

1. Preheat your oven to 375°F (190°C).

2. In a bowl, whisk together the eggs, milk, salt, and pepper.

3. Grease a muffin tin with cooking oil or butter.

4. Distribute the chopped mixed vegetables evenly among the muffin cups.

5. Pour the egg mixture over the vegetables, filling each cup about 3/4 full.

6. Sprinkle the shredded cheese on top of each muffin cup.

7. Bake in the preheated oven for approximately 15-20 minutes or until the egg muffins are set and slightly golden on top.

8. Remove from the oven and allow them to cool for a few minutes before removing them from the muffin tin.

9. Serve these delicious egg and vegetable muffins as a convenient and protein-packed breakfast option.

Blueberry Chia Pudding

Ingredients:

- 1/4 cup chia seeds
- 1 cup low-fat milk (dairy or non-dairy)

- 1 tablespoon honey or maple syrup
- 1/2 teaspoon vanilla extract
- 1/4 cup fresh or frozen blueberries

Instructions:

1. In a jar or bowl, combine the chia seeds, low-fat milk, honey or maple syrup, and vanilla extract. Stir well to combine.
2. Let the mixture sit for a few minutes, then stir again to prevent clumping.
3. Cover the jar or bowl and refrigerate overnight or for at least 4 hours to allow the chia seeds to absorb the liquid and create a pudding-like consistency.
4. Before serving, give the chia pudding a good stir to evenly distribute the seeds.
5. Top the pudding with fresh or frozen blueberries for a burst of fruity flavor.
6. Enjoy the creamy and nutritious blueberry chia pudding as a delightful breakfast treat.

Rice Porridge with Raisins

Ingredients:

- 1/2 cup cooked white rice
- 1 cup water or milk (dairy or non-dairy)
- 2 tablespoons raisins
- 1 tablespoon honey or maple syrup (optional)
- 1/4 teaspoon cinnamon

Instructions:

1. In a small saucepan, combine the cooked white rice, water or milk, and raisins.
2. Bring the mixture to a boil over medium heat, stirring occasionally.
3. Reduce the heat to low and simmer for about 10 minutes or until the porridge reaches your desired consistency, stirring occasionally.
4. Remove the saucepan from heat and stir in honey or maple syrup if desired.
5. Sprinkle cinnamon on top of the rice porridge for a warm and comforting aroma.
6. Let the porridge cool slightly before enjoying this nourishing and easy-to-digest breakfast option.

Chapter 3: Lunch Recipes

These lunch recipes are designed for a low-fiber diet, which may be recommended for individuals with diverticulitis.

Chicken and Vegetable Stir-Fry

Ingredients:

- 2 boneless, skinless chicken breasts, thinly sliced
- 1 tablespoon vegetable oil
- 2 cloves garlic, minced
- 1 red bell pepper, sliced
- 1 yellow bell pepper, sliced
- 1 small broccoli crown, cut into florets
- 1 medium carrot, julienned
- 1/4 cup low-sodium soy sauce
- 1 tablespoon honey
- 1 teaspoon cornstarch
- Salt and pepper, to taste
- Sesame seeds, for garnish (optional)

Instructions:

1. In a small bowl, whisk together soy sauce, honey, and cornstarch. Set aside.

2. Heat vegetable oil in a large skillet or wok over medium-high heat.

3. Add minced garlic and sauté for 1 minute until fragrant.

4. Add chicken slices to the skillet and stir-fry until cooked through, about 5-6 minutes. Remove from skillet and set aside.

5. In the same skillet, add the sliced bell peppers, broccoli florets, and julienned carrot. Stir-fry for 4-5 minutes until vegetables are crisp-tender.

6. Return the cooked chicken to the skillet and pour the soy sauce mixture over the ingredients. Stir well to coat everything evenly.

7. Cook for an additional 2-3 minutes until the sauce thickens slightly.

8. Season with salt and pepper to taste.

9. Serve the chicken and vegetable stir-fry hot, garnished with sesame seeds if desired. Enjoy!

Turkey and Avocado Wrap

Ingredients:

- 4 whole wheat tortillas
- 8 ounces cooked turkey breast, sliced
- 1 avocado, peeled, pitted, and sliced
- 1 cup baby spinach leaves
- 1/4 cup sliced red onion
- 2 tablespoons plain Greek yogurt
- 1 tablespoon Dijon mustard
- Salt and pepper, to taste

Instructions:

1. Lay out the whole wheat tortillas on a clean surface.
2. In a small bowl, mix together Greek yogurt and Dijon mustard. Spread the mixture evenly on each tortilla.
3. Layer the sliced turkey, avocado, baby spinach, and red onion on top of the tortillas.
4. Season with salt and pepper to taste.
5. Roll up the tortillas tightly, tucking in the sides as you go.

6. Cut the wraps in half diagonally and secure with toothpicks if necessary.

7. Serve the turkey and avocado wraps immediately or wrap them in plastic wrap for later. Enjoy!

Tuna Salad Lettuce Wraps

Ingredients:

- 2 cans tuna, drained
- 1/4 cup mayonnaise
- 2 tablespoons diced red onion
- 2 tablespoons diced celery
- 2 tablespoons diced pickles
- 1 tablespoon lemon juice
- Salt and pepper, to taste
- Lettuce leaves, for wrapping

Instructions:

1. In a medium bowl, combine tuna, mayonnaise, red onion, celery, pickles, and lemon juice.

2. Mix well until all ingredients are evenly coated.

3. Season with salt and pepper to taste.

4. Place a spoonful of the tuna salad onto a lettuce leaf.

5. Fold the sides of the lettuce leaf over the filling and roll it up tightly.

6. Repeat with the remaining lettuce leaves and tuna salad.

7. Serve the tuna salad lettuce wraps as a refreshing and light lunch option. Enjoy!

Shrimp and Quinoa Salad

Ingredients:

- 1 cup cooked quinoa
- 1 pound shrimp, peeled and deveined
- 1 tablespoon olive oil
- 1 clove garlic, minced
- 1/2 teaspoon paprika
- Salt and pepper, to taste
- 1 cup cherry tomatoes, halved
- 1 cucumber, diced
- 1/4 cup chopped fresh parsley
- Juice of 1 lemon

Instructions:

1. In a large skillet, heat olive oil over medium heat.
2. Add minced garlic and sauté for 1 minute until fragrant.
3. Add the shrimp to the skillet and sprinkle with paprika, salt, and pepper.
4. Cook the shrimp for 2-3 minutes per side until pink and cooked through.
5. In a large bowl, combine cooked quinoa, cherry tomatoes, diced cucumber, chopped parsley, and the cooked shrimp.
6. Squeeze the lemon juice over the salad and toss everything together to combine.
7. Adjust seasoning with salt and pepper if needed.
8. Serve the shrimp and quinoa salad chilled or at room temperature. Enjoy!

Baked Salmon with Lemon and Herbs

Ingredients:

- 4 salmon fillets
- 2 tablespoons olive oil

- 2 cloves garlic, minced
- Zest of 1 lemon
- Juice of 1 lemon
- 1 teaspoon dried dill
- Salt and pepper, to taste

Instructions:

1. Preheat the oven to 375°F (190°C) and line a baking sheet with parchment paper.
2. Place the salmon fillets on the prepared baking sheet.
3. In a small bowl, whisk together olive oil, minced garlic, lemon zest, lemon juice, dried dill, salt, and pepper.
4. Brush the lemon and herb mixture over the salmon fillets, coating them evenly.
5. Bake the salmon for 12-15 minutes until it flakes easily with a fork and is cooked to your desired doneness.
6. Remove the salmon from the oven and let it rest for a few minutes before serving.

7. Serve the baked salmon with lemon and herbs hot, garnished with additional lemon slices if desired. Enjoy!

Egg Salad with Greek Yogurt

Ingredients:

- 6 hard-boiled eggs, peeled and chopped
- 1/4 cup plain Greek yogurt
- 1 tablespoon Dijon mustard
- 2 tablespoons chopped fresh dill
- 2 tablespoons chopped fresh chives
- Salt and pepper, to taste
- Whole grain bread or lettuce leaves, for serving

Instructions:

1. In a medium bowl, combine chopped hard-boiled eggs, Greek yogurt, Dijon mustard, chopped dill, and chopped chives.
2. Mix well until all ingredients are evenly combined.
3. Season with salt and pepper to taste.

4. Serve the egg salad on whole grain bread as a sandwich or wrap it in lettuce leaves for a low-carb option.

5. Enjoy the creamy and flavorful egg salad with Greek yogurt for a satisfying lunch.

Lentil Soup with Carrots and Celery

Ingredients:

- 1 cup dried lentils, rinsed and drained
- 1 tablespoon olive oil
- 1 onion, chopped
- 2 cloves garlic, minced
- 2 carrots, diced
- 2 celery stalks, diced
- 4 cups vegetable broth
- 1 teaspoon dried thyme
- 1 bay leaf
- Salt and pepper, to taste
- Fresh parsley, for garnish (optional)

Instructions:

1. Heat olive oil in a large pot over medium heat.

2. Add chopped onion, minced garlic, diced carrots, and diced celery to the pot. Sauté for 5-6 minutes until vegetables soften.

3. Add rinsed lentils, vegetable broth, dried thyme, bay leaf, salt, and pepper to the pot.

4. Bring the mixture to a boil, then reduce heat to low and simmer for 30-35 minutes until lentils are tender.

5. Remove the bay leaf from the soup and discard.

6. Using an immersion blender or a countertop blender, blend the soup until smooth and creamy.

7. If using a countertop blender, return the blended soup to the pot.

8. Adjust seasoning with salt and pepper if needed.

9. Serve the lentil soup with carrots and celery hot, garnished with fresh parsley if desired. Enjoy!

Greek Salad with Grilled Chicken

Ingredients:

- 2 boneless, skinless chicken breasts
- 1 tablespoon olive oil
- 1 teaspoon dried oregano

- Salt and pepper, to taste
- 4 cups chopped romaine lettuce
- 1 cup cherry tomatoes, halved
- 1 cucumber, diced
- 1/2 red onion, thinly sliced
- 1/2 cup pitted Kalamata olives
- 1/2 cup crumbled feta cheese
- Juice of 1 lemon
- 2 tablespoons extra virgin olive oil

Instructions:

1. Preheat a grill or grill pan over medium-high heat.
2. Season the chicken breasts with olive oil, dried oregano, salt, and pepper.
3. Grill the chicken for 6-8 minutes per side until cooked through. Remove from heat and let it rest for a few minutes before slicing.
4. In a large bowl, combine chopped romaine lettuce, cherry tomatoes, diced cucumber, sliced red onion, Kalamata olives, and crumbled feta cheese.
5. In a small bowl, whisk together lemon juice and extra virgin olive oil to make the dressing.

6. Drizzle the dressing over the salad ingredients and toss everything together to combine.

7. Slice the grilled chicken and arrange it on top of the Greek salad.

8. Serve the Greek salad with grilled chicken as a fresh and hearty lunch option. Enjoy!

Zucchini Noodles with Tomato Sauce

Ingredients:

- 4 medium zucchini
- 2 tablespoons olive oil
- 2 cloves garlic, minced
- 1 can (14 ounces) diced tomatoes
- 1 teaspoon dried basil
- 1/2 teaspoon dried oregano
- Salt and pepper, to taste
- Grated Parmesan cheese, for garnish (optional)

Instructions:

1. Trim the ends of the zucchini and spiralize them into noodles using a spiralizer.

2. Heat olive oil in a large skillet over medium heat.

3. Add minced garlic to the skillet and sauté for 1 minute until fragrant.

4. Add the spiralized zucchini noodles to the skillet and cook for 2-3 minutes until they are slightly softened but still retain a bit of crunch.

5. In a separate saucepan, combine diced tomatoes, dried basil, dried oregano, salt, and pepper. Cook over medium heat for 5-6 minutes until the sauce thickens slightly.

6. Pour the tomato sauce over the zucchini noodles in the skillet and toss everything together to coat the noodles evenly.

7. Cook for an additional 2-3 minutes until the noodles are heated through.

8. Serve the zucchini noodles with tomato sauce hot, garnished with grated Parmesan cheese if desired. Enjoy!

Roasted Vegetable and Quinoa Salad

Ingredients:

- 1 cup cooked quinoa
- 1 small eggplant, diced
- 1 zucchini, diced
- 1 red bell pepper, diced
- 1 yellow bell pepper, diced
- 1 red onion, thinly sliced
- 2 tablespoons olive oil
- 1 teaspoon dried thyme
- Salt and pepper, to taste
- Juice of 1 lemon
- 2 tablespoons chopped fresh parsley

Instructions:

1. Preheat the oven to 425°F (220°C) and line a baking sheet with parchment paper.
2. In a large bowl, combine diced eggplant, diced zucchini, diced red bell pepper, diced yellow bell pepper, and thinly sliced red onion.
3. Drizzle olive oil over the vegetables and sprinkle with dried thyme, salt, and pepper. Toss everything together to coat the vegetables evenly.

4. Spread the seasoned vegetables in a single layer on the prepared baking sheet.

5. Roast the vegetables in the preheated oven for 20-25 minutes until they are tender and lightly browned, stirring once halfway through.

6. In a large bowl, combine cooked quinoa, roasted vegetables, lemon juice, and chopped parsley. Toss everything together to combine.

7. Adjust seasoning with salt and pepper if needed.

8. Serve the roasted vegetable and quinoa salad as a satisfying and nutritious lunch option. Enjoy!

Chapter 4: Dinner Recipes

In this chapter, we will explore a variety of delicious dinner recipes that are suitable for a low fiber diet, perfect for individuals with diverticulitis. These recipes are not only nutritious but also packed with flavor, ensuring that you can enjoy a satisfying and wholesome meal while following your dietary restrictions.

Grilled Chicken Breast with Steamed Vegetables

Ingredients:

- 4 boneless, skinless chicken breasts
- 1 tablespoon olive oil
- Salt and pepper, to taste
- 1 teaspoon garlic powder
- 1 teaspoon paprika
- 2 cups mixed vegetables (broccoli, carrots, cauliflower)
- Lemon wedges, for serving

Instructions:

1. Preheat the grill to medium-high heat.
2. Brush the chicken breasts with olive oil and season them with salt, pepper, garlic powder, and paprika.
3. Place the chicken breasts on the grill and cook for 6-8 minutes per side, or until the internal temperature reaches 165°F (74°C).
4. While the chicken is grilling, steam the mixed vegetables until tender-crisp.
5. Serve the grilled chicken breasts with steamed vegetables and lemon wedges on the side.

Baked Cod with Herbed Quinoa

Ingredients:

- 4 cod fillets
- 2 tablespoons lemon juice
- 2 tablespoons olive oil
- 1 teaspoon dried oregano
- 1 teaspoon dried thyme
- Salt and pepper, to taste
- 1 cup quinoa
- 2 cups vegetable broth

- Chopped fresh parsley, for garnish

Instructions:

1. Preheat the oven to 400°F (200°C).
2. Place the cod fillets in a baking dish and drizzle them with lemon juice and olive oil. Sprinkle with dried oregano, dried thyme, salt, and pepper.
3. Bake the cod in the preheated oven for 12-15 minutes, or until it flakes easily with a fork.
4. Meanwhile, rinse the quinoa under cold water and drain well.
5. In a saucepan, combine the quinoa and vegetable broth. Bring to a boil, then reduce the heat, cover, and simmer for about 15 minutes, or until the liquid is absorbed and the quinoa is tender.
6. Fluff the cooked quinoa with a fork and stir in chopped fresh parsley.
7. Serve the baked cod over a bed of herbed quinoa.

Beef and Broccoli Stir-Fry

Ingredients:

- 1 lb beef sirloin, thinly sliced

- 2 tablespoons soy sauce

- 1 tablespoon cornstarch

- 2 tablespoons vegetable oil

- 2 cloves garlic, minced

- 1 teaspoon grated fresh ginger

- 2 cups broccoli florets

- 1 red bell pepper, sliced

- 1/4 cup low-sodium beef broth

- 2 tablespoons oyster sauce

- Cooked rice, for serving

Instructions:

1. In a bowl, combine the sliced beef, soy sauce, and cornstarch. Toss to coat the beef evenly and set aside.

2. Heat the vegetable oil in a large skillet or wok over high heat.

3. Add the minced garlic and grated ginger to the hot oil and stir-fry for about 30 seconds.

4. Add the beef to the skillet and stir-fry for 2-3 minutes, until browned.

5. Add the broccoli florets and sliced bell pepper to the skillet and stir-fry for an additional 2-3 minutes, until the vegetables are crisp-tender.

6. In a small bowl, whisk together the beef broth and oyster sauce. Pour the mixture into the skillet and stir-fry for another minute.

7. Serve the beef and broccoli stir-fry over cooked rice.

Turkey Meatballs with Marinara Sauce

Ingredients:

- 1 lb ground turkey
- 1/2 cup breadcrumbs
- 1/4 cup grated Parmesan cheese
- 1/4 cup chopped fresh parsley
- 1 egg
- 2 cloves garlic, minced
- 1 teaspoon dried basil
- 1/2 teaspoon dried oregano
- Salt and pepper, to taste
- 2 cups marinara sauce

Instructions:

1. Preheat the oven to 375°F (190°C).

2. In a large bowl, combine the ground turkey, breadcrumbs, Parmesan cheese, chopped parsley, egg, minced garlic, dried basil, dried oregano, salt, and pepper. Mix well.

3. Shape the mixture into meatballs, about 1 inch in diameter, and place them on a baking sheet lined with parchment paper.

4. Bake the meatballs in the preheated oven for 20-25 minutes, or until they are cooked through and browned.

5. In a saucepan, heat the marinara sauce over medium heat until warmed.

6. Add the cooked meatballs to the marinara sauce and simmer for 5 minutes.

7. Serve the turkey meatballs with marinara sauce over pasta or zucchini noodles.

Stuffed Bell Peppers with Ground Turkey

Ingredients:

- 4 bell peppers (any color)
- 1 lb ground turkey
- 1 small onion, chopped
- 2 cloves garlic, minced
- 1 cup cooked quinoa
- 1 cup marinara sauce
- 1 teaspoon dried basil
- 1 teaspoon dried oregano
- Salt and pepper, to taste
- Shredded mozzarella cheese, for topping

Instructions:

1. Preheat the oven to 375°F (190°C).
2. Cut off the tops of the bell peppers and remove the seeds and membranes. Place the peppers upright in a baking dish.
3. In a skillet, cook the ground turkey, chopped onion, and minced garlic over medium heat until the turkey is browned and the onion is softened.

4. Add the cooked quinoa, marinara sauce, dried basil, dried oregano, salt, and pepper to the skillet. Stir well to combine.

5. Spoon the turkey and quinoa mixture into the bell peppers, filling them to the top.

6. Cover the baking dish with foil and bake in the preheated oven for 25-30 minutes.

7. Remove the foil, sprinkle the stuffed peppers with shredded mozzarella cheese, and bake for an additional 5 minutes, or until the cheese is melted and bubbly.

8. Serve the stuffed bell peppers with ground turkey as a satisfying main dish.

Lemon Herb Roasted Chicken Thighs

Ingredients:

- 4 bone-in, skin-on chicken thighs
- 2 tablespoons olive oil
- 2 tablespoons lemon juice
- 2 cloves garlic, minced
- 1 teaspoon dried thyme
- 1 teaspoon dried rosemary

- Salt and pepper, to taste
- Lemon slices, for garnish
- Fresh parsley, for garnish

Instructions:

1. Preheat the oven to 425°F (220°C).
2. In a small bowl, whisk together the olive oil, lemon juice, minced garlic, dried thyme, dried rosemary, salt, and pepper.
3. Place the chicken thighs in a baking dish and pour the lemon herb marinade over them, turning to coat evenly.
4. Arrange lemon slices on top of the chicken thighs.
5. Roast the chicken in the preheated oven for 30-35 minutes, or until the chicken reaches an internal temperature of 165°F (74°C) and the skin is golden brown and crispy.
6. Garnish with fresh parsley and serve the lemon herb roasted chicken thighs with your choice of side dishes.

Shrimp Scampi with Zucchini Noodles

Ingredients:

- 1 lb shrimp, peeled and deveined
- 2 tablespoons butter
- 2 tablespoons olive oil
- 4 cloves garlic, minced
- 1/2 teaspoon red pepper flakes (optional)
- Juice of 1 lemon
- Salt and pepper, to taste
- 4 medium zucchini, spiralized into noodles
- Chopped fresh parsley, for garnish

Instructions:

1. In a large skillet, melt the butter with the olive oil over medium heat.
2. Add the minced garlic and red pepper flakes (if using) to the skillet and sauté for 1 minute, until fragrant.
3. Add the shrimp to the skillet and cook for 2-3 minutes on each side, until pink and cooked through.

4. Squeeze the lemon juice over the shrimp and season with salt and pepper to taste.

5. Remove the shrimp from the skillet and set aside.

6. In the same skillet, add the zucchini noodles and sauté for 2-3 minutes, until they are slightly softened.

7. Return the cooked shrimp to the skillet and toss to combine with the zucchini noodles.

8. Garnish with chopped fresh parsley and serve the shrimp scampi with zucchini noodles as a light and flavorful dinner option.

Vegetable Curry with Brown Rice

Ingredients:

- 1 tablespoon vegetable oil
- 1 onion, chopped
- 2 cloves garlic, minced
- 1 tablespoon curry powder
- 1 teaspoon ground cumin
- 1/2 teaspoon ground turmeric
- 1/4 teaspoon cayenne pepper (optional, for heat)

- 2 cups mixed vegetables (carrots, peas, bell peppers, cauliflower)
- 1 can (14 oz) coconut milk
- 1 cup vegetable broth
- Salt and pepper, to taste
- Cooked brown rice, for serving

Instructions:

1. Heat the vegetable oil in a large saucepan or skillet over medium heat.
2. Add the chopped onion and minced garlic to the pan and sauté for 2-3 minutes, until softened.
3. Stir in the curry powder, ground cumin, ground turmeric, and cayenne pepper (if using), and cook for another minute to toast the spices.
4. Add the mixed vegetables to the pan and cook for 3-4 minutes, until they begin to soften.
5. Pour in the coconut milk and vegetable broth, and season with salt and pepper to taste. Stir well to combine.

6. Simmer the vegetable curry over low heat for 15-20
    minutes, until the vegetables are tender and the
    flavors are well blended.
7. Serve the vegetable curry over cooked brown rice
    for a satisfying and nourishing dinner.

Pork Tenderloin with Roasted Vegetables

Ingredients:

- 1 lb pork tenderloin
- 2 tablespoons olive oil, divided
- 2 cloves garlic, minced
- 1 teaspoon dried thyme
- 1 teaspoon dried rosemary
- Salt and pepper, to taste
- 2 cups mixed root vegetables (carrots, potatoes, parsnips)
- 1 red onion, sliced
- 1 tablespoon balsamic vinegar
- Chopped fresh parsley, for garnish

Instructions:

1. Preheat the oven to 400°F (200°C).

2. Rub the pork tenderloin with 1 tablespoon of olive oil, minced garlic, dried thyme, dried rosemary, salt, and pepper.

3. Heat the remaining 1 tablespoon of olive oil in a large oven-safe skillet over medium-high heat.

4. Sear the pork tenderloin in the hot skillet for 2-3 minutes on each side, until browned.

5. Transfer the skillet with the pork tenderloin to the preheated oven and roast for 20-25 minutes, or until the pork reaches an internal temperature of 145°F (63°C).

6. While the pork is roasting, prepare the roasted vegetables. Toss the mixed root vegetables and sliced red onion with balsamic vinegar, salt, and pepper.

7. Spread the vegetables on a baking sheet and roast in the oven for 20-25 minutes, or until tender and caramelized.

8. Let the pork tenderloin rest for a few minutes before slicing. Garnish with chopped fresh parsley and serve with the roasted vegetables.

Teriyaki Tofu Stir-Fry

Ingredients:

- 1 lb firm tofu, drained and cut into cubes
- 2 tablespoons soy sauce
- 2 tablespoons teriyaki sauce
- 1 tablespoon rice vinegar
- 1 tablespoon honey (or maple syrup for a vegan option)
- 1 tablespoon vegetable oil
- 2 cloves garlic, minced
- 1 teaspoon grated fresh ginger
- 2 cups mixed stir-fry vegetables (broccoli, bell peppers, snap peas)
- Cooked brown rice, for serving

Instructions:

1. In a bowl, whisk together the soy sauce, teriyaki sauce, rice vinegar, and honey (or maple syrup). Set aside.
2. Heat the vegetable oil in a large skillet or wok over medium-high heat.

3. Add the minced garlic and grated ginger to the hot oil and stir-fry for about 30 seconds.

4. Add the tofu cubes to the skillet and cook for 4-5 minutes, until lightly browned.

5. Pour the teriyaki sauce mixture over the tofu and stir to coat.

6. Add the mixed stir-fry vegetables to the skillet and stir-fry for an additional 3-4 minutes, until the vegetables are crisp-tender.

7. Serve the teriyaki tofu stir-fry over cooked brown rice for a flavorful and satisfying dinner.

Chapter 5: Snacks and Appetizers

In this chapter, we will explore a variety of delicious snacks and appetizers that are perfect for those following a low fiber diet. These recipes are not only tasty but also easy to prepare. Let's dive into the world of flavorful treats that will satisfy your cravings while keeping your digestive system happy.

Greek Yogurt Dip with Fresh Veggies

Ingredients:

- 1 cup Greek yogurt
- 1 tablespoon lemon juice
- 1 clove garlic, minced
- 1 teaspoon dried dill
- Salt and pepper to taste
- Assorted fresh vegetables (carrots, cucumbers, bell peppers, cherry tomatoes, etc.)

Instructions:

1. In a bowl, combine the Greek yogurt, lemon juice, minced garlic, dried dill, salt, and pepper. Mix well until all the ingredients are thoroughly combined.

2. Taste the dip and adjust the seasoning according to your preference.

3. Wash and cut the fresh vegetables into bite-sized pieces for dipping.

4. Serve the Greek yogurt dip with the assorted fresh vegetables and enjoy a refreshing and healthy snack.

Avocado Hummus with Rice Crackers

Ingredients:

- 1 ripe avocado, peeled and pitted
- 1 cup canned chickpeas, drained and rinsed
- 2 tablespoons tahini
- 2 tablespoons lemon juice
- 1 clove garlic, minced
- 1/4 teaspoon ground cumin
- Salt and pepper to taste
- Rice crackers for serving

Instructions:

1. In a food processor, combine the avocado, chickpeas, tahini, lemon juice, minced garlic, ground cumin, salt, and pepper. Blend until smooth and creamy.

2. Taste the hummus and adjust the seasoning if needed.

3. Transfer the avocado hummus to a serving bowl and garnish with a drizzle of olive oil and a sprinkle of paprika, if desired.

4. Serve the avocado hummus with rice crackers and enjoy a delectable and nutritious snack.

Baked Sweet Potato Fries

Ingredients:

- 2 large sweet potatoes, peeled and cut into fries
- 2 tablespoons olive oil
- 1 teaspoon paprika
- 1/2 teaspoon garlic powder
- Salt and pepper to taste

Instructions:

1. Preheat the oven to 425°F (220°C) and line a baking sheet with parchment paper.
2. In a large bowl, combine the sweet potato fries, olive oil, paprika, garlic powder, salt, and pepper. Toss until the fries are evenly coated with the seasonings.
3. Arrange the sweet potato fries in a single layer on the prepared baking sheet.
4. Bake for 20-25 minutes, or until the fries are crispy and golden brown, flipping them halfway through the cooking time for even browning.
5. Remove the baked sweet potato fries from the oven and let them cool for a few minutes before serving. Enjoy these guilt-free fries as a delightful snack or appetizer.

Caprese Skewers with Balsamic Glaze

Ingredients:

*   Cherry tomatoes
*   Fresh mozzarella cheese, cut into bite-sized pieces

- Fresh basil leaves
- Balsamic glaze

Instructions:

1. Thread a cherry tomato onto a skewer, followed by a piece of mozzarella cheese and a fresh basil leaf.
2. Repeat the process until you have assembled all the caprese skewers.
3. Arrange the skewers on a serving platter.
4. Drizzle balsamic glaze over the caprese skewers just before serving.
5. These elegant and flavorful skewers make a perfect addition to any party or gathering.

Deviled Eggs with Pickles

Ingredients:

- 6 hard-boiled eggs, peeled
- 3 tablespoons mayonnaise
- 1 tablespoon Dijon mustard
- 1 tablespoon pickle relish
- Salt and pepper to taste
- Paprika for garnish

Instructions:

1. Slice the hard-boiled eggs in half lengthwise and carefully remove the yolks.

2. In a bowl, mash the egg yolks using a fork.

3. Add mayonnaise, Dijon mustard, pickle relish, salt, and pepper to the mashed egg yolks. Mix until well combined and creamy.

4. Spoon the deviled egg mixture back into the egg white halves, dividing it evenly.

5. Sprinkle paprika over the deviled eggs for an added touch of flavor and presentation.

6. Chill the deviled eggs in the refrigerator for at least 30 minutes before serving. These tangy and savory bites are a classic favorite for any occasion.

Guacamole with Carrot Sticks

Ingredients:

- 2 ripe avocados, peeled and pitted
- 1/2 red onion, finely chopped
- 1 small tomato, diced
- 1 jalapeño pepper, seeded and minced (optional)

- 1 tablespoon lime juice
- 1 clove garlic, minced
- Salt and pepper to taste
- Carrot sticks for serving

Instructions:

1. In a bowl, mash the avocados using a fork until desired consistency is reached.
2. Add the finely chopped red onion, diced tomato, minced jalapeño pepper (if using), lime juice, minced garlic, salt, and pepper. Mix well to combine all the ingredients.
3. Taste the guacamole and adjust the seasoning according to your preference.
4. Transfer the guacamole to a serving bowl and garnish with a sprinkle of chopped cilantro, if desired.
5. Serve the guacamole with carrot sticks and enjoy a zesty and nutritious snack.

Roasted Chickpeas with Herbs

Ingredients:

- 1 can chickpeas, drained and rinsed
- 2 tablespoons olive oil
- 1 teaspoon dried oregano
- 1/2 teaspoon paprika
- 1/4 teaspoon garlic powder
- Salt and pepper to taste

Instructions:

1. Preheat the oven to 400°F (200°C) and line a baking sheet with parchment paper.
2. Rinse the chickpeas thoroughly and pat them dry with a clean towel or paper towel.
3. In a bowl, toss the chickpeas with olive oil, dried oregano, paprika, garlic powder, salt, and pepper until they are well coated with the seasonings.
4. Spread the seasoned chickpeas in a single layer on the prepared baking sheet.
5. Roast the chickpeas in the preheated oven for 20-25 minutes, or until they become crispy and golden brown, shaking the baking sheet occasionally for even cooking.

6. Remove the roasted chickpeas from the oven and let them cool before serving. These crunchy and protein-packed snacks are sure to be a hit.

Spinach and Artichoke Dip

Ingredients:

- 1 cup frozen spinach, thawed and drained
- 1 cup canned artichoke hearts, drained and chopped
- 1 cup Greek yogurt
- 1/2 cup grated Parmesan cheese
- 1/2 cup shredded mozzarella cheese
- 1/4 cup mayonnaise
- 1 clove garlic, minced
- Salt and pepper to taste
- Tortilla chips or pita bread for serving

Instructions:

1. Preheat the oven to 375°F (190°C).
2. In a bowl, combine the thawed and drained spinach, chopped artichoke hearts, Greek yogurt, grated Parmesan cheese, shredded mozzarella cheese, mayonnaise, minced garlic, salt, and pepper. Mix

well until all the ingredients are evenly incorporated.

3. Transfer the spinach and artichoke dip mixture to a baking dish.

4. Bake in the preheated oven for 20-25 minutes, or until the dip is bubbly and lightly browned on top.

5. Remove the dip from the oven and let it cool for a few minutes before serving.

6. Serve the spinach and artichoke dip with tortilla chips or pita bread for a warm and creamy appetizer.

Cucumber and Cream Cheese Roll-Ups

Ingredients:

- 1 large cucumber
- 4 ounces cream cheese, softened
- 1 tablespoon chopped fresh dill
- 1 tablespoon chopped fresh chives
- Salt and pepper to taste

Instructions:

1. Peel the cucumber and cut it lengthwise into thin slices using a mandoline or a sharp knife.

2. In a small bowl, mix together the softened cream cheese, chopped fresh dill, chopped fresh chives, salt, and pepper until well combined.

3. Place a cucumber slice on a flat surface and spread a thin layer of the cream cheese mixture on top.

4. Roll up the cucumber slice tightly and secure it with a toothpick.

5. Repeat the process with the remaining cucumber slices and cream cheese mixture.

6. Chill the cucumber and cream cheese roll-ups in the refrigerator for at least 30 minutes before serving. These refreshing and creamy bites make a delightful addition to any party or gathering.

Sliced Apple with Almond Butter

Ingredients:

- Apples, cored and sliced
- Almond butter

Instructions:

1. Slice the apples into thin rounds or wedges.

2. Spread a generous amount of almond butter on each apple slice.

3. Arrange the sliced apples on a platter or serve them individually.

4. Enjoy the perfect combination of crisp sweetness from the apples and creamy nuttiness from the almond butter.

Chapter 6: Desserts

In this chapter, we will explore a variety of delicious desserts that are suitable for a low fiber diet. These desserts are not only satisfying but also packed with flavor and nutrition. From fruity delights to creamy indulgences, these desserts will surely satisfy your sweet tooth without compromising your dietary restrictions. Let's dive into the wonderful world of low fiber desserts!

Banana "Ice Cream" with Almonds

Ingredients:

- 2 ripe bananas
- 1/4 cup chopped almonds

Instructions:

1. Peel the bananas and cut them into small chunks.
2. Place the banana chunks in a freezer bag and freeze them for at least 2 hours or until they are completely frozen.

3. Once frozen, transfer the banana chunks to a blender or food processor.

4. Blend the frozen bananas until they turn into a smooth and creamy consistency, resembling soft serve ice cream.

5. Scoop the banana "ice cream" into serving bowls.

6. Sprinkle the chopped almonds on top.

7. Serve immediately and enjoy this guilt-free frozen treat!

Baked Apples with Cinnamon and Yogurt

Ingredients:

- 4 medium-sized apples
- 1 tablespoon honey
- 1 teaspoon ground cinnamon
- 1/2 cup plain Greek yogurt

Instructions:

1. Preheat your oven to 350°F (175°C).

2. Core the apples using an apple corer or a small knife, removing the seeds and stem.

3. Place the cored apples in a baking dish.

4. Drizzle the honey over the apples, ensuring they are evenly coated.

5. Sprinkle the ground cinnamon over the honey-coated apples.

6. Bake the apples in the preheated oven for about 30 minutes or until they are tender.

7. Once baked, remove the apples from the oven and let them cool slightly.

8. Serve each baked apple with a dollop of Greek yogurt on top.

9. Sprinkle some additional cinnamon if desired.

10. Enjoy the warm, comforting flavors of this delightful dessert!

Chocolate Avocado Pudding

Ingredients:

- 2 ripe avocados
- 1/4 cup unsweetened cocoa powder
- 1/4 cup honey or maple syrup
- 1/2 teaspoon vanilla extract
- Pinch of salt

- Optional toppings: chopped nuts, berries, or shredded coconut

Instructions:

1. Cut the avocados in half, remove the pits, and scoop the flesh into a blender or food processor.
2. Add the cocoa powder, honey or maple syrup, vanilla extract, and salt to the blender.
3. Blend the mixture until smooth and creamy, scraping down the sides as needed.
4. Taste the pudding and adjust the sweetness if desired by adding more honey or maple syrup.
5. Once the desired consistency and sweetness are achieved, transfer the pudding to serving bowls.
6. Refrigerate the pudding for at least 30 minutes to allow it to set.
7. Before serving, garnish with your choice of chopped nuts, berries, or shredded coconut.
8. Indulge in this rich and decadent chocolate pudding that's surprisingly healthy!

Berry Parfait with Greek Yogurt

Ingredients:

- 1 cup mixed berries (strawberries, blueberries, raspberries)
- 1 cup plain Greek yogurt
- 1 tablespoon honey
- 1/4 cup granola (optional)

Instructions:

1. Wash the berries and pat them dry with a paper towel.
2. In a bowl, mix the Greek yogurt and honey until well combined.
3. In serving glasses or bowls, layer the Greek yogurt mixture, followed by a layer of mixed berries.
4. Repeat the layers until the glasses or bowls are filled.
5. Top each parfait with a sprinkle of granola for added crunch (optional).
6. Serve immediately or refrigerate until ready to serve.

7. Enjoy the refreshing combination of creamy yogurt and juicy berries in this delightful parfait!

Coconut Macaroons

Ingredients:

- 2 cups unsweetened shredded coconut
- 3/4 cup sweetened condensed milk
- 1 teaspoon vanilla extract
- Pinch of salt
- Optional: melted dark chocolate for drizzling (optional)

Instructions:

1. Preheat your oven to 325°F (163°C) and line a baking sheet with parchment paper.
2. In a bowl, combine the shredded coconut, sweetened condensed milk, vanilla extract, and salt.
3. Stir the mixture until all the ingredients are well incorporated.
4. Using a cookie scoop or your hands, scoop out portions of the mixture and shape them into small mounds.

5. Place the coconut mounds on the prepared baking sheet, spacing them evenly apart.

6. Bake the macaroons in the preheated oven for about 20 minutes or until they turn golden brown.

7. Once baked, remove the macaroons from the oven and let them cool completely.

8. Optional: If desired, drizzle melted dark chocolate over the cooled macaroons for an extra touch of decadence.

9. Allow the chocolate to set before serving or storing the macaroons.

10. Enjoy these delightful coconut treats that are chewy on the inside and crispy on the outside!

Chia Seed Pudding with Mango

Ingredients:

- 1/4 cup chia seeds
- 1 cup unsweetened almond milk (or any milk of your choice)
- 1 tablespoon honey or maple syrup
- 1/2 teaspoon vanilla extract
- 1 ripe mango, diced

Instructions:

1. In a bowl, combine the chia seeds, almond milk, honey or maple syrup, and vanilla extract.

2. Stir the mixture until the chia seeds are evenly distributed.

3. Let the mixture sit for about 5 minutes, then stir again to prevent clumping.

4. Cover the bowl and refrigerate the mixture for at least 2 hours or overnight to allow it to thicken.

5. Once the chia seed pudding has thickened to your desired consistency, remove it from the refrigerator.

6. Give it a good stir and divide the pudding into serving glasses or bowls.

7. Top each serving with diced mango.

8. Serve chilled and savor the creamy texture and fruity sweetness of this chia seed pudding!

Poached Pears with Honey and Cinnamon

Ingredients:

*   4 ripe pears
*   2 cups water

- 1/4 cup honey

- 1 cinnamon stick

- 1 teaspoon lemon juice

- Optional: Greek yogurt or vanilla ice cream for serving

Instructions:

1. Peel the pears, leaving the stems intact.

2. In a saucepan, combine the water, honey, cinnamon stick, and lemon juice.

3. Bring the mixture to a simmer over medium heat, stirring to dissolve the honey.

4. Add the peeled pears to the simmering liquid and cook for about 15-20 minutes or until the pears are tender.

5. Remove the poached pears from the liquid and let them cool slightly.

6. Serve the poached pears on individual plates or bowls.

7. Optionally, serve with a dollop of Greek yogurt or a scoop of vanilla ice cream for added creaminess.

8. Drizzle some of the poaching liquid over the pears as a sweet sauce.

9. Delight in the fragrant and tender poached pears, complemented by the comforting flavors of honey and cinnamon.

Lemon Bars with Almond Flour Crust

Ingredients:

For the crust:

- 1 1/2 cups almond flour
- 1/4 cup melted coconut oil
- 2 tablespoons honey or maple syrup
- Pinch of salt

For the lemon filling:

- 4 large eggs
- 3/4 cup fresh lemon juice
- 1/2 cup honey or maple syrup
- 2 tablespoons almond flour
- 1 tablespoon lemon zest

Instructions:

1. Preheat your oven to 350°F (175°C) and line an 8x8-inch baking pan with parchment paper.
2. In a bowl, combine the almond flour, melted coconut oil, honey or maple syrup, and salt for the crust.
3. Stir the mixture until it forms a crumbly dough.
4. Press the dough evenly into the bottom of the prepared baking pan.
5. Bake the crust in the preheated oven for about 10 minutes or until it turns golden brown.
6. While the crust is baking, prepare the lemon filling.
7. In another bowl, whisk together the eggs, lemon juice, honey or maple syrup, almond flour, and lemon zest until well combined.
8. Once the crust is done baking, pour the lemon filling over the hot crust.
9. Return the pan to the oven and bake for an additional 15-20 minutes or until the filling is set.
10. Remove the pan from the oven and let it cool completely before slicing into bars.

11. Refrigerate the lemon bars for a few hours to allow
    them to chill and firm up.

12. Enjoy these tangy and zesty lemon bars with their
    delightful almond flour crust!

Pumpkin Muffins with Walnuts

Ingredients:

- 1 3/4 cups almond flour
- 1/4 cup coconut flour
- 1 teaspoon baking powder
- 1/2 teaspoon baking soda
- 1/2 teaspoon ground cinnamon
- 1/4 teaspoon ground nutmeg
- 1/4 teaspoon ground ginger
- Pinch of salt
- 1 cup canned pumpkin puree
- 1/4 cup honey or maple syrup
- 3 large eggs
- 1/4 cup melted coconut oil
- 1 teaspoon vanilla extract
- 1/2 cup chopped walnuts

Instructions:

1. Preheat your oven to 350°F (175°C) and line a muffin tin with paper liners.
2. In a large bowl, whisk together the almond flour, coconut flour, baking powder, baking soda, ground cinnamon, ground nutmeg, ground ginger, and salt.
3. In a separate bowl, combine the pumpkin puree, honey or maple syrup, eggs, melted coconut oil, and vanilla extract.
4. Add the wet ingredients to the dry ingredients and mix until well combined.
5. Fold in the chopped walnuts.
6. Spoon the batter into the prepared muffin tin, filling each liner about 3/4 full.
7. Bake the muffins in the preheated oven for 20-25 minutes or until a toothpick inserted into the center comes out clean.
8. Once baked, remove the muffins from the oven and let them cool in the tin for a few minutes.
9. Transfer the muffins to a wire rack to cool completely before enjoying.

10. These moist and flavorful pumpkin muffins with a delightful crunch from the walnuts are perfect for a cozy treat!

Grilled Pineapple with Coconut Whipped Cream

Ingredients:

- 1 ripe pineapple
- 1/2 cup coconut cream
- 1 tablespoon honey or maple syrup
- 1/2 teaspoon vanilla extract

Instructions:

1. Preheat your grill to medium-high heat.
2. Peel the pineapple and cut it into rings or spears, discarding the core.
3. Place the pineapple slices on the preheated grill and cook for about 2-3 minutes on each side or until they develop grill marks.
4. While the pineapple is grilling, prepare the coconut whipped cream.

5. In a mixing bowl, combine the coconut cream, honey or maple syrup, and vanilla extract.

6. Whip the mixture with an electric mixer on medium speed until it reaches a creamy and fluffy consistency.

7. Remove the grilled pineapple from the grill and let it cool slightly.

8. Serve the grilled pineapple with a dollop of coconut whipped cream on top.

9. Optionally, garnish with a sprinkle of shredded coconut for added tropical flair.

10. Indulge in the smoky-sweet flavors of the grilled pineapple paired with the creamy and luscious coconut whipped cream.

Chapter 7: Smoothies

Smoothies are a delicious and refreshing way to incorporate healthy ingredients into your diet. In this chapter, we will explore ten different smoothie recipes that are not only packed with flavor but also provide essential nutrients to support your well-being. Whether you're looking for a burst of energy in the morning or a refreshing pick-me-up in the afternoon, these smoothies will satisfy your taste buds and nourish your body.

Berry Blast Smoothie

Ingredients:

- 1 cup mixed berries (strawberries, blueberries, raspberries)
- 1 ripe banana
- 1 cup almond milk
- 1 tablespoon honey
- 1 tablespoon chia seeds
- Ice cubes (optional)

Instructions:

1. Wash the berries thoroughly and remove any stems.

2. Peel the banana and break it into chunks.

3. Place the berries, banana, almond milk, honey, and chia seeds in a blender.

4. Blend on high speed until the mixture is smooth and creamy.

5. If desired, add a few ice cubes and blend again to make it colder.

6. Pour the smoothie into a glass and enjoy immediately.

Tropical Green Smoothie

Ingredients:

- 1 cup fresh spinach
- 1 ripe mango, peeled and pitted
- 1 ripe banana
- 1 cup coconut water
- 1 tablespoon lime juice
- 1 tablespoon flaxseeds
- Ice cubes (optional)

Instructions:

1. Rinse the spinach leaves thoroughly.

2. Cut the mango and banana into chunks.

3. In a blender, combine the spinach, mango, banana, coconut water, lime juice, and flaxseeds.

4. Blend on high speed until the mixture becomes smooth and creamy.

5. If desired, add a few ice cubes and blend again for a colder smoothie.

6. Pour the tropical green smoothie into a glass and enjoy its refreshing flavors.

Banana and Peanut Butter Smoothie

Ingredients:

- 2 ripe bananas
- 2 tablespoons peanut butter
- 1 cup almond milk
- 1 tablespoon honey
- 1/2 teaspoon vanilla extract
- Ice cubes (optional)

Instructions:

1. Peel the bananas and break them into chunks.

2. In a blender, combine the banana chunks, peanut butter, almond milk, honey, and vanilla extract.

3. Blend on high speed until the mixture is smooth and creamy.

4. If desired, add a few ice cubes and blend again for a chilled texture.

5. Pour the banana and peanut butter smoothie into a glass and savor its delightful taste.

Spinach and Mango Smoothie

Ingredients:

- 2 cups fresh spinach
- 1 ripe mango, peeled and pitted
- 1 cup pineapple chunks
- 1/2 cup orange juice
- 1/2 cup Greek yogurt
- Ice cubes (optional)

Instructions:

1. Wash the spinach leaves thoroughly.

2. Cut the mango into chunks and discard the pit.

3. In a blender, combine the spinach, mango chunks, pineapple chunks, orange juice, and Greek yogurt.

4. Blend on high speed until the mixture becomes smooth and creamy.

5. If desired, add a few ice cubes and blend again for a chilled smoothie.

6. Pour the spinach and mango smoothie into a glass and enjoy its vibrant flavors.

Chocolate Banana Protein Smoothie

Ingredients:

- 1 ripe banana
- 1 cup almond milk
- 1 tablespoon cocoa powder
- 1 tablespoon honey
- 1 scoop chocolate protein powder
- Ice cubes (optional)

Instructions:

1. Peel the banana and break it into chunks.

2. In a blender, combine the banana chunks, almond milk, cocoa powder, honey, and chocolate protein powder.

3. Blend on high speed until the mixture is well blended and creamy.

4. If desired, add a few ice cubes and blend again for a colder smoothie.

5. Pour the chocolate banana protein smoothie into a glass and indulge in its rich and satisfying taste.

Blueberry and Almond Smoothie

Ingredients:

- 1 cup blueberries
- 1 ripe banana
- 1 cup almond milk
- 1 tablespoon almond butter
- 1 tablespoon honey
- Ice cubes (optional)

Instructions:

1. Wash the blueberries thoroughly.

2. Peel the banana and break it into chunks.

3. In a blender, combine the blueberries, banana chunks, almond milk, almond butter, and honey.

4. Blend on high speed until the mixture becomes smooth and creamy.

5. If desired, add a few ice cubes and blend again for a chilled smoothie.

6. Pour the blueberry and almond smoothie into a glass and relish its delightful combination.

Avocado and Spinach Smoothie

Ingredients:

- 1 ripe avocado
- 2 cups fresh spinach
- 1 cup coconut water
- 1 tablespoon lime juice
- 1 tablespoon honey
- Ice cubes (optional)

Instructions:

1. Cut the avocado in half, remove the pit, and scoop out the flesh.

2. Rinse the spinach leaves thoroughly.

3. In a blender, combine the avocado flesh, spinach leaves, coconut water, lime juice, and honey.

4. Blend on high speed until the mixture becomes smooth and creamy.

5. If desired, add a few ice cubes and blend again for a colder smoothie.

6. Pour the avocado and spinach smoothie into a glass and enjoy its creamy texture and nourishing properties.

Pineapple and Coconut Smoothie

Ingredients:

- 1 cup pineapple chunks
- 1/2 cup coconut milk
- 1/2 cup Greek yogurt
- 1 tablespoon honey
- 1/2 teaspoon vanilla extract
- Ice cubes (optional)

Instructions:

1.   In a blender, combine the pineapple chunks,
     coconut milk, Greek yogurt, honey, and vanilla
     extract.
2.   Blend on high speed until the mixture becomes
     smooth and creamy.
3.   If desired, add a few ice cubes and blend again for a
     chilled smoothie.
4.   Pour the pineapple and coconut smoothie into a
     glass and indulge in its tropical flavors.

Strawberry and Oat Smoothie

Ingredients:

*   1 cup fresh strawberries
*   1 ripe banana
*   1/2 cup rolled oats
*   1 cup almond milk
*   1 tablespoon honey
*   Ice cubes (optional)

Instructions:

1.   Rinse the strawberries thoroughly and remove the
     stems.

2. Peel the banana and break it into chunks.

3. In a blender, combine the strawberries, banana chunks, rolled oats, almond milk, and honey.

4. Blend on high speed until the mixture becomes smooth and creamy.

5. If desired, add a few ice cubes and blend again for a colder smoothie.

6. Pour the strawberry and oat smoothie into a glass and savor its fruity and satisfying taste.

Peach and Greek Yogurt Smoothie

Ingredients:

- 2 ripe peaches, pitted and sliced
- 1/2 cup Greek yogurt
- 1 cup almond milk
- 1 tablespoon honey
- 1/2 teaspoon vanilla extract
- Ice cubes (optional)

Instructions:

1. In a blender, combine the peach slices, Greek yogurt, almond milk, honey, and vanilla extract.

2. Blend on high speed until the mixture becomes smooth and creamy.

3. If desired, add a few ice cubes and blend again for a chilled smoothie.

4. Pour the peach and Greek yogurt smoothie into a glass and enjoy its luscious and refreshing flavor.

CONCLUSION

As we reach the culmination of our journey through the Low Fiber Diet Cookbook for Diverticulitis. Throughout this cookbook, we have explored various aspects of diverticulitis and how a low fiber diet can play a crucial role in managing the condition. Now, as we wrap up our exploration, let us recap the key points, discuss the importance of maintaining a low fiber diet for long-term health, and offer some final thoughts and encouragement.

Recap of Key Points

Throughout this cookbook, we have emphasized the importance of understanding diverticulitis and the role of a low fiber diet in its management. We delved into the definition of diverticulitis and provided insights into how it affects the digestive system. We discussed the benefits of a low fiber diet, such as reducing strain on the colon and minimizing the risk of complications. Additionally, we provided practical tips for following a low fiber diet effectively.

In the 30 Day Meal Plan, we presented a comprehensive guide for individuals looking to embark on a low fiber diet journey. We organized meal plans and recipes for four weeks, offering a variety of delicious and nutritious options to ensure that individuals can enjoy their meals while adhering to the dietary restrictions. The accompanying grocery lists were designed to simplify the shopping experience and aid in planning the meals.

We then proceeded to explore breakfast, lunch, dinner, snacks, appetizers, desserts, and smoothie recipes specifically tailored for a low fiber diet. These recipes were carefully crafted to be both satisfying and flavorful, ensuring that individuals with diverticulitis can still enjoy a diverse range of meals while adhering to their dietary requirements.

Maintaining a Low Fiber Diet for Long-Term Health
While this cookbook has provided you with a wealth of information and delicious recipes, it is essential to recognize that a low fiber diet should not be seen as a

temporary measure solely for managing diverticulitis flare-ups. Rather, it can form the foundation of a long-term approach to maintaining gut health and overall well-being.

To effectively maintain a low fiber diet for long-term health, it is crucial to work in collaboration with your healthcare provider or a registered dietitian. They can provide personalized guidance based on your specific needs, ensuring that you meet all your nutritional requirements while managing diverticulitis effectively.

In addition to following a low fiber diet, it is essential to adopt other healthy lifestyle practices. Regular exercise, stress management techniques, and staying hydrated are all crucial components of maintaining optimal gut health. Furthermore, it is important to maintain a balanced and varied diet that includes a wide range of nutrients to support overall wellness.

Final Thoughts and Encouragement

Embarking on a low fiber diet for diverticulitis can initially feel overwhelming. It requires making adjustments to your eating habits, exploring new recipes, and staying committed to your health. However, it is important to remember that you are not alone in this journey. There are countless individuals who have successfully managed diverticulitis through dietary modifications.

As you conclude this cookbook, I encourage you to approach your low fiber diet with a positive mindset. Embrace the opportunity to discover new flavors, experiment with different ingredients, and find joy in preparing meals that support your well-being. Remember to seek support from loved ones and connect with online communities or support groups where you can share experiences and learn from others facing similar challenges.

Lastly, always remember that your health is a top priority. Stay in regular contact with your healthcare provider, schedule routine check-ups, and discuss any concerns or questions you may have. By being proactive and informed, you can ensure that you are on the right track to managing diverticulitis effectively.